Understanding cervical smear...

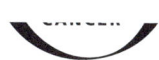

This booklet is for you if you have had, or are about to have, a cervical smear test. Your doctor or nurse may wish to go through the booklet with you and mark sections that are particularly important for you. You can make a note below of the main contacts and information that you may need quickly.

Specialist nurse/contact names ....

....

....

Hospital

Phone ....

Treatments ....

....

....

....

Family doctor ....

....

....

Surgery address

If you like you can also add:

Your name ....

Address. ....

....

Understanding cervical smears

This booklet aims to tell you about cervical smears. These two pages sum up the main points, and show which pages to turn to for more information.

The smear test Page 8

The smear test is a simple, quick procedure. It can be slightly uncomfortable but should not be painful.

The doctor or nurse takes a sample of cells from the cervix. The cells are spread onto a glass slide and sent to a laboratory for examination under a microscope.

What is an abnormal smear? Page 9

The smear test is the routine test for detecting early changes in the cells of the cervix. The medical name for these changes is **CIN** (cervical intra-epithelial neoplasia). There are three categories of CIN – 1 (mild), 2 (moderate) and 3 (severe).

These abnormal cells are **not** cancerous but if left untreated they can sometimes go on to develop into cancer of the cervix.

What causes CIN? Pages 11-12

The exact cause of CIN is still unknown. It does appear to be related to sexual activity, and there is also thought to be a link with a number of sexually transmitted viruses. Women who smoke are more likely to develop CIN than women who do not.

Further tests Pages 13-14

Many abnormal smears showing borderline or mild changes will return to normal on their own, so your doctor may simply arrange for you to have another smear test in a few months.

Key points in this booklet

If your smear shows moderate or severe changes, your doctor may suggest you have further tests straight away and will refer you for colposcopy.

What treatments are used for CIN? Page 15

Treatments which can be used for CIN include:

- laser therapy
- cryotherapy
- cold coagulation
- diathermy
- cone biopsy
- large loop excision of the transformation zone (LLETZ)

These treatments are almost 100% successful in eliminating the condition, but it may sometimes recur.

Your feelings Page 18

You may feel frightened or uncertain if you have been told that you have an abnormal smear. However, there is no need to feel like this, or to worry in silence. There are many people available to help you: your GP or practice nurse and, if you have any treatment, the doctor and nurses at the hospital where you receive it. Do not be afraid to ask them about anything that you don't understand or that is worrying you.

For more information

There are other ways to obtain information. This booklet lists useful organisations (pages 20-21), books that might help (page 22), and BACUP's booklets (page 23).

The nurses in BACUP's Cancer Information Service (0171 613 2121 or Freephone 0800 18 11 99) can give information about all aspects of cancer, and people who can help.

If you need to talk through your feelings in depth, you can contact BACUP's Cancer Counselling Service on 0171 696 9000, or at BACUP Scotland in Glasgow on 0141 553 1553.

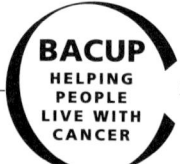 3 Bath Place, Rivington Street, London, EC2A 3JR

BACUP was founded by Dr Vicky Clement-Jones, following her own experiences with ovarian cancer, and offers information, counselling and support to people with cancer, their families and friends.

We produce publications on the main types of cancer, treatments, and ways of living with cancer. We also produce a magazine, *BACUP News,* three times a year.

Our success depends on feedback from users of the service. We thank everyone, particularly patients and their families, whose advice has made this booklet possible.

Administration 0171 696 9003
Cancer Information Service 0171 613 2121 (8 lines)
Freeline 0800 18 11 99
Cancer Counselling Service 0171 696 9000 (London)
BACUP Scotland Cancer Counselling Service
0141 553 1553 (Glasgow)

British Association of Cancer United Patients and their families and friends. A company limited by guarantee. Registered in England and Wales company number 2803321. Charity registration number 1019719. Registered office 3 Bath Place, Rivington Street, London, EC2A 3JR

Medical consultant: Dr Maurice Slevin, MD, FRCP

Editor: Stella Wood

Illustrations: Mark de Pienne

Cover design: Alison Hooper Associates

This revised edition published 1997

© BACUP 1988, 1991, 1997

All rights reserved. No part of this publication may be reproduced or transmitted, in any form or by any means, electronic or mechanical, including photocopying, recording or any information storage and retrieval system, without permission in writing from BACUP.

Typeset and printed in Great Britain by Lithoflow Ltd., London

ISBN 1-870403-95-9

Contents

Introduction	6
The cervix	7
Cervical screening	8
Where to go for your smear test	8
The smear test	8
Cervical erosion or ectopy	9
What is an abnormal smear?	9
The grades of CIN	11
What causes CIN?	11
What are the symptoms of CIN?	12
Further tests	13
Colposcopy	13
Cone biopsy	14
What treatments are used for CIN?	15
How are the treatments given?	16
Laser therapy	16
Cryotherapy	16
Cold coagulation	16
Diathermy	17
Cone biopsy	17
Large loop excision of the transformation zone (LLETZ)	17
Hysterectomy	17
Your feelings	18
BACUP's services	19
Useful organisations	20
Books recommended by BACUP	22
BACUP booklets	23
Questions you might like to ask your doctor (fill-in page)	*facing inside back cover*

Introduction

This information booklet has been written to help you understand what is meant by a cervical smear and what happens if an 'abnormal smear' is discovered.

We hope it answers some of the questions you may have about abnormal smears and their treatment.

We can't advise you about the best treatment for yourself because this information can only come from your own doctor who will be familiar with your full medical history.

At the end of this booklet you will find a list of other BACUP publications, some useful addresses and recommended books, and a page to fill in with any questions you may have for your doctor. If, after reading this booklet, you think it has helped you, do pass it on to any of your family and friends who might find it interesting. They too may want to be informed so they can help you cope with any problems you may have.

The cervix

The cervix is the lower part of the uterus, or womb. Sometimes it is also called the neck of the womb. The uterus is a muscular, pear-shaped organ at the top of the vagina. The lining of the uterus is shed each month, giving rise to bleeding called a period. These periods stop temporarily during pregnancy and will normally continue until a woman has the menopause.

It is possible for your doctor to see and feel the cervix during an internal (vaginal) examination.

The surface layer of the cervix is made up of two different types of cells, flat cells called squamous cells and tall cells called columnar cells. The place where these two cells meet is known as the transformation zone. It is in this area that abnormal cell changes occur. It is these cells, on the surface of the cervix, which are examined in a cervical smear test.

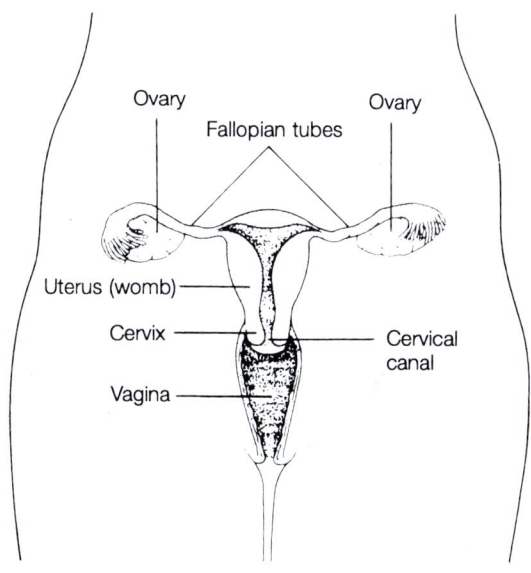

The position of the cervix

Cervical screening

Under the present Department of Health guidelines women between the ages of 20 and 64 should have a cervical smear test at least every five years. However, many health authorities call and recall women every three years. Women who have had previous treatment for CIN may need a smear test more frequently. Your doctor will discuss this with you.

Where to go for your smear test

Most women go to their GP for their smear test but tests are also done at Family Planning and Well Woman clinics as well as genito-urinary clinics (see list of Useful Organisations on page 21).

When you make an appointment for a smear test try to make sure that it is in the middle of your menstrual cycle (about half-way between one period and the next).

The smear test

The smear test is a very simple test and takes less than five minutes. It can be slightly uncomfortable but should not be painful.

Once you are lying comfortably on the couch the doctor or nurse will gently insert an instrument called a speculum to keep the vagina open. A small spatula is then used to take a sample of cells from the cervix. The cells are spread onto a glass slide and sent to a laboratory for examination under a microscope.

After you have had your smear test you may like to ask your doctor how long it will take for the results to come back. The NHS Cervical Screening Programme recommends four weeks as a reasonable time.

If you do not hear anything from your GP after this time, give the surgery or health centre a ring and ask them to check up on your results.

If the results show that abnormal cells are present, your doctor will contact you and either arrange a second smear test or refer you to a doctor who specialises in women's health (gynaecologist).

> **Remember – most women with an abnormal smear do not have cancer of the cervix**

Cervical erosion or ectopy

During your smear test your doctor may notice that you have a condition known as a 'cervical erosion' or 'ectopy'. This is where the squamous cells on the surface of the cervix are replaced by columnar cells and the cervix may look inflamed.

This condition is very common, particularly during puberty and pregnancy and in women who are taking the pill. A cervical erosion is completely harmless and is in no way associated with CIN or cancer of the cervix. It may occasionally cause bleeding or discharge, particularly after sex, in which case it can be easily treated. If an erosion has occurred during pregnancy, it usually returns to normal by itself, or it can easily be treated once the baby is born.

What is an abnormal smear?

The smear, or Pap test, as it is sometimes called, is the routine test for detecting early changes in the cells of the cervix. The medical name for these changes is CIN, which stands for cervical intra-epithelial neoplasia. The changes may also be referred to as dyskaryosis. All this means is that when the cells are looked at under a microscope they are abnormal.

> **These abnormal cells are not cancerous but if left untreated they can sometimes go on to develop into cancer of the cervix**

For this reason they are also known as pre-cancerous changes. If these early changes are detected on your smear test, it is known as an abnormal smear.

Occasionally changes to the glandular cells which line the cervical canal (endocervix) may be detected on a cervical smear test.

Changes to these cells seem to go through the same process as with CIN but would be reported as CGIN, which stands for cervical glandular intra-epithelial neoplasia.

A form of cervical cancer called adenocarcinoma may arise from these changed glandular cells. If abnormal glandular cells are detected on a smear test, then further investigations would be undertaken.

A cervical smear can also detect cancer of the cervix but most women with an abnormal smear have early cell changes and not cancer.

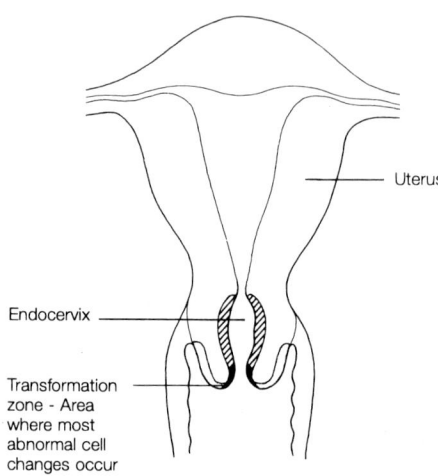

Sometimes your doctor may ask you to have another smear because the specimen taken was 'inadequate'. This means that not enough cells were collected at your first test, or the test was otherwise unreadable.

Some test results may be 'borderline' or show mild changes only. This means that there are slight cell changes on the cervix, which may revert to normal. Further monitoring will be needed, but not necessarily any treatment.

If your test result is borderline, you will need to have another smear. If the changes remain, your doctor may recommend that you visit a gynaecologist for further tests.

The grades of CIN

When the abnormal cells are looked at under a microscope they are divided into three categories. This makes it easier for the doctor to decide on the best form of treatment for you.

CIN 1 – only one third of the thickness of the covering layer of the cervix is affected.

CIN 2 – two thirds of the thickness of the covering layer of the cervix is affected.

CIN 3 – the full thickness of the covering layer of the cervix is affected.

With all three grades of CIN, often only a small part of the cervix is affected by abnormal changes.

CIN 3 is also known as carcinoma-in-situ. Although this sounds like cancer, CIN 3 is **not** cancer of the cervix. However, it is important that it is treated as soon as possible. It is only when the cells below the surface layer of the cervix are penetrated that cancer of the cervix has developed. BACUP has a booklet called *Understanding cancer of the cervix* which we would be happy to send you if it is appropriate.

What causes CIN?

The exact cause of CIN is still unknown. It does appear to be related to sexual activity and is commoner in women who became sexually active at a young age. There is also thought to be a link with a number of viruses, for example the human papilloma virus (HPV). As these viruses are sexually transmitted, the possibility of developing the virus increases with the number of partners a woman or her partner has had.

This link between CIN and sex has resulted in many women blaming themselves, or their partners, for causing it. However, sex is only one of the many factors associated with CIN, and only a small proportion of women with any of the known risk factors will develop CIN.

There is evidence that barrier methods of contraception, such as the cap or condoms, act as a protection against the spread of the viruses linked with CIN.

Some evidence suggests that there is an increased risk of developing cancer of the cervix if women have taken the contraceptive pill for more than ten years. However, it is still unclear whether this is due to the contraceptive pill itself or to other factors. If you are concerned about taking the contraceptive pill, please discuss it with your GP or local family planning service.

Women who smoke are more likely to develop CIN than non-smokers. Research has suggested that some substance in cigarette smoke, when it is inhaled and absorbed into the bloodstream, may affect certain immune cells in the cervix which protect against papilloma viruses. Once these cells are weakened, the cervix is more vulnerable to the effect of these viruses.

What are the symptoms of CIN?

Most women with CIN do not have any symptoms at all. Occasionally, it may show as irregular bleeding from the vagina, especially after sex, and as new bleeding in women who have already had the menopause.

Irregular bleeding is common to many conditions other than CIN. It is very important that you always have it checked by your doctor.

As most women do not have any symptoms it is essential to have regular smear tests to detect any early cell changes (see page 8 for details about the smear test).

Further tests

Many abnormal smears showing borderline or mild changes will return to normal on their own, so your doctor may simply arrange for you to have a further smear test in a few months. If your second smear still shows abnormal cells, your doctor may arrange for you to have some further tests.

With moderate or severe changes, your doctor may suggest you have further tests right away. These tests include any of the following:

Colposcopy

This is a closer examination of the abnormal areas using a colposcope, which is like a small microscope. The colposcope acts like a magnifying glass so the doctor can see the whole cervix in more detail. Colposcopy is usually done at a hospital out-patients clinic. Some hospitals do not have the facilities for colposcopy and you may have to go to a more specialised hospital in your area.

Before your test the nurse will help you to position yourself on the couch. When you are lying comfortably the doctor will use a speculum, in the same way as the smear test, to hold the vagina open. The cervix is then painted with a solution to make the abnormal areas show up more clearly. A light is shone onto the cervix and the doctor will look through a colposcope to examine the surface of the cervix in more detail. A small sample of tissue (biopsy) is taken from the cervix for examination under a microscope.

Colposcopy takes a bit longer than the smear test, usually about 10-15 minutes. In general it is not painful, but it may be uncomfortable.

If the abnormal area still can't be seen clearly with a colposcope, your doctor may arrange for you to have a cone biopsy.

Cone biopsy

This is done while you are under a general anaesthetic and will mean a short stay in hospital.

While you are under the anaesthetic the doctor takes a small cone-shaped section of the abnormal tissue from the cervix for examination under a microscope.

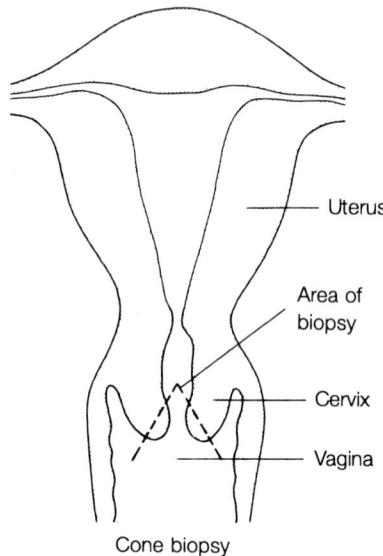

Cone biopsy

After your operation a small pack of gauze may be put into the vagina (like a tampon) to prevent bleeding. This is usually removed within 24 hours.

It is normal to have some light bleeding and discharge for a few days after your operation. Strenuous physical activity and sex should be avoided for at least four weeks to allow the cervix to heal properly.

Occasionally a cone biopsy can lead to a weakening of the cervix, which may increase the risk of miscarriage during pregnancy. This can usually be prevented by inserting a stitch into the cervix to strengthen it during pregnancy. Your doctor will discuss this with you in more detail. A cone biopsy will in no way affect your ability to enjoy sex or to get pregnant.

What treatments are used for CIN?

Sometimes the cells showing CIN 1 will return to normal without any treatment at all. If your doctor decides not to treat these minor changes, regular smears should be taken to ensure that further cell changes do not take place. Some doctors prefer to treat any abnormality, however mild.

The main treatments that are used for CIN are laser therapy, cryotherapy, cold coagulation, diathermy, cone biopsy and large loop excision of the transformation zone (LLETZ). All these treatments are very successful and most women only need to have one session of treatment. The type of treatment you have will depend upon a number of factors. These will include the facilities which are available at your local hospital and the type of treatment which your doctor feels would be most appropriate for you.

Laser therapy, cryotherapy and cold coagulation are usually given in a hospital out-patient clinic. Some women feel slightly unwell for a few hours after their treatment and it is a good idea to arrange to have the day off work.

Diathermy and cone biopsy are done under a general anaesthetic and will mean a short stay in hospital.

Your doctor will probably advise you not to have sex, or use tampons, for at least three to four weeks after your treatment to allow the cervix to heal properly. After any treatment for CIN you will need extra follow up for the next five years to check that the treatment has been successful. The form that the follow up takes will vary from hospital to hospital.

Treatments for CIN will NOT have any effect on your ability to enjoy sex or to get pregnant (unless you choose to have a hysterectomy (which is extremely rare) – see page 17), once the cervix has healed.

How are the treatments given?

Most women only need one of the treatments described on these pages.

Before your treatment the nurse will help you position yourself on the couch. The doctor will then use a speculum to hold the vagina open, in the same way as a smear test.

Try to relax as much as possible and don't be afraid to ask the doctor or nurse as many questions as you like about your treatment. The treatment itself usually takes about five to ten minutes and although it may be slightly uncomfortable it is not painful.

Laser therapy

Once you are lying comfortably on the couch the doctor will put some local anaesthetic onto the cervix to numb it. A laser beam is then pointed onto the abnormal areas of the cervix and the cells are destroyed. During the treatment you may notice a slight burning smell from the laser. This is quite normal.

Most women have some light bleeding and discharge after laser treatment. If the bleeding gets heavier you should contact your GP or the out-patient department where you had your treatment.

Cryotherapy

Once you are lying comfortably on the couch the doctor will gently place a small probe onto the surface of the cervix to freeze the abnormal cells. During the treatment you may feel a mild period-type pain but this will disappear once the treatment has finished.

It is normal to have a watery vaginal discharge for about two to three weeks after cryotherapy.

Cold coagulation

Despite the name of this treatment the cells are removed by heating not freezing. This is done by placing a hot probe onto the surface of the cervix. You will not be able to feel this although you may have a mild period-type pain during your treatment.

There are not usually any side effects after cold coagulation although some women may have light bleeding for a couple of days.

Diathermy

While you are under a general anaesthetic the doctor destroys the abnormal cells by passing a tiny electrical current through the affected area. Diathermy is very quick and you will probably be back on the ward in less than an hour.

Some women have a slight vaginal discharge or bleeding like a light period, for a few days after their treatment.

Cone biopsy

Cone biopsy was discussed on page 14 as a way of diagnosing CIN if the abnormal area cannot be seen clearly with a colposcope. It can also be used as a form of treatment for CIN. A small, cone-shaped piece of cervix, which contains the abnormal cells, is removed while you are under a general anaesthetic.

Large loop excision of the transformation zone (LLETZ)

This is often used instead of a cone biopsy, but is carried out under local anaesthetic and uses a thin wire to cut through the affected area. You may experience some discomfort, but this varies from woman to woman.

Hysterectomy

In women who are past childbearing age or who have completed their families an operation to remove the womb (hysterectomy) is sometimes done for CIN.

For women who have not yet had the menopause the ovaries will not be removed with the womb, so this treatment will not bring on an early menopause.

If you do find that you have any problem after your treatment, don't be afraid to go back to your doctor. And remember BACUP's specialist cancer nurses are always happy to discuss any problems with you.

Your feelings

When a woman is told that she has an abnormal smear her first reaction is often one of fear. Many women immediately think that they have cancer. Although the smear test is also used to check for cancer of the cervix the vast majority of women who have an abnormal smear have early changes in the cells and do **not** have cancer.

Recently there has been a lot of publicity about CIN and its link with sex and sexually transmitted diseases. This has led to many women feeling guilty or ashamed if they have been told they have CIN. It seems to be true that the more partners you have, the more likely you are to contract the human papilloma virus, which is thought to be linked with the development of CIN.

However, many women with CIN have only had one sexual partner, and only a small proportion of women who have any of the known risk factors will develop CIN.

Many women find the treatments for CIN embarrassing and frightening. They sometimes react by becoming tense, tearful or withdrawn. Don't be afraid to ask the doctor or nurses as many questions as you like, as this may help to put your mind at rest. The BACUP nurses are also happy to answer any of your questions. Some women like to take their partner or a close friend with them when they have treatment, others prefer to 'go it alone'.

Research has shown that the treatments for CIN are very successful and do not usually need repeating. Women who have had successful treatment for an abnormal smear are also very unlikely to have a recurrence of the problem.

BACUP's services

Cancer Information Service

If, after reading this booklet, you have any questions about cervical smears, further tests or CIN and its treatments, please contact BACUP's Cancer Information Service and speak to one of our experienced cancer nurses. The Cancer Information Service is open to telephone enquiries from 9am to 7pm Monday to Friday.

The number to call is: 0171 613 2121. You can call the Cancer Information Service free of charge on 0800 18 11 99.

Alternatively you can write to us at 3 Bath Place, Rivington Street, London EC2A 3JR.

Cancer Counselling Service

BACUP's Cancer Counselling Service can give information about local counselling services and can discuss with people whether counselling could be appropriate and helpful for them. BACUP runs a one-to-one counselling service based at its London and Glasgow offices.

For more information about counselling, or to make an appointment with BACUP's Cancer Counselling Service, please ring 0171 696 9000 (London) or 0141 553 1553 (Glasgow).

Useful organisations

BACUP
3 Bath Place
Rivington Street
London
EC2A 3JR
Office: 0171 696 9003

BACUP Scotland
Cancer Counselling Service
30 Bell Street
Glasgow
G1 1LG
Office: 0141 553 1553

Cancer Information Service
0171 613 2121 or Freephone: 0800 18 11 99
Open 9am-7pm Monday to Friday.

Cancer Counselling Service
London: 0171 696 9000
Glasgow: 0141 553 1553
All BACUP's London numbers can take minicom calls.

Jersey BACUP
6 Royal Crescent, St Helier, Jersey JE2 4QG
Tel: 01534 89904 Freephone: 1200 275
In addition to providing a link with BACUP's Cancer Information Service in the Channel Islands, Jersey BACUP runs a local cancer support group and trained local volunteers give support over the telephone, and in the local hospital.

Family Planning Association (FPA)
2-12 Pentonville Road, London N1 9FP
Tel: 0171 837 5432
Provides free information about family planning, contraceptives and sexual health.

Women's Health Information Centre
52 Featherstone Street, London EC1Y 8RT
Tel: 0171 251 6580
Information and leaflets about all aspects of women's health in English and some Asian languages. Provides contact with other women who have had abnormal smears.

Women's Nationwide Cancer Control Campaign (WNCCC)
Suna House, 128-130 Curtain Road, London EC2A 3AR
Tel: 0171 729 4688
     0171 729 2229 (helpline, Mon-Fri 9.30am-4.30pm)
Offers information and advice on cervical screening.

Details of Family Planning, Well Woman and genito-urinary clinics can be found in your local phone directory or at your doctor's surgery or local health centre.

Books recommended by BACUP

Anne Szarewski
A woman's guide to the cervical smear test
Optima, 1994
ISBN 0-3562-1033-2   £6.99

Explains what a smear test is and how it is carried out. Discusses abnormal smears and the treatments that may be given. Section on emotions and reactions to having a smear test. Useful illustrations.

Sally Haslett
Having a cervical smear
Beaconsfield Publishers, 1994
ISBN 0-9065-8438-8   £2.50

Question and answer format. Discusses what the test involves, the different investigations and treatments and explains technical terms.

BACUP booklets

Understanding cancer series:

Acute lymphoblastic leukaemia
Acute myeloblastic leukaemia
Bladder
Bone cancer – primary
Bone cancer – secondary
Brain tumours
Breast – primary
Breast – secondary
Cervical smears
Cervix
Chronic lymphocytic leukaemia
Chronic myeloid leukaemia
Colon and rectum
Hodgkin's disease
Kaposi's sarcoma
Kidney
Larynx
Liver
Lung
Lymphoedema
Malignant melanoma
Mouth and throat
Myeloma
Non-Hodgkin's lymphoma
Oesophagus
Ovary
Pancreas
Prostate
Skin
Soft tissue sarcomas
Stomach
Testes
Thyroid
Uterus
Vulva

Understanding treatment series:

Bone marrow and stem cell transplants
Breast reconstruction
Chemotherapy
Clinical trials
Radiotherapy
Tamoxifen factsheet

Living with cancer series:

Complementary therapies and cancer
Coping at home: caring for someone with advanced cancer
Coping with hair loss
Diet and the cancer patient
Facing the challenge of advanced cancer
Feeling better: controlling pain and other symptoms of cancer
Lost for words: how to talk to someone with cancer
Sexuality and cancer
What do I tell the children? – a guide for a parent with cancer
What now? Adjusting to life after cancer
Who can ever understand? – talking about your cancer
Will power – a step-by-step guide to making or changing your will

Questions you might like to ask your doctor or surgeon

You can fill this in before you see the doctor or surgeon, and then use it to remind yourself of the questions you want to ask, and the answers you receive.

1. ....

Answer ....

....

2. ....

Answer ....

....

3. ....

Answer ....

....

4. ....

Answer ....

....

5. ....

Answer ....

....

6. ....

Answer ....

....